Essential Oil Beauty Secrets

ADISH Books

Copyright © 2013 ADISH Books

ISBN: 1491244933

ISBN-13: 978-1491244937

Text Copyright © 2013 ADISH Books

Disclaimer

The information specified throughout this book is provided for general information only, and should not be treated as a substitute for the medical advice of your own doctor, psychiatrist, medical counsellor or any other health care professional. Nothing contained on this book is intended to be for medical diagnosis or treatment. By following the instructions contained herein, the reader willingly assumes all risks in connection with such instructions. If you think you have a medical emergency, call your doctor immediately.

Preface

This book provides comprehensive information of commonly used essential oils in beauty products and explains how essential oils can play a crucial role in our daily regimen, ranging from hair care to nail care.

We are living in a world full of chemicals. We use chemical products from morning until night. From toothpaste in the morning to makeup cleaner at night, all are chemical products in a cosmetic world.

Nature didn't design our bodies to absorb all these chemicals. Our body is accumulating toxic materials day by day and these foreign materials are harming our body because our body doesn't know what to do with them. What is the solution? We need to give our body some breathing space by reducing the rate of chemical injection in it. This would allow it to start its inherent purification process to remove these toxic materials. We cannot remove all these materials from our life immediately without having proper replacements for them, but we can try to make an honest difference for our bodies. We can begin the long journey of detoxifying the body in small steps, starting with our outer self. By replacing our chemical cosmetics with the natural products, you will be on the road to cleansing your body and allowing it to heal.

This book provides you with details of chemical-free recipes and natural alternatives to potentially harmful hair and skin care products. You will gain an understanding of how the anti-bacterial properties in essential oils work to treat numerous skin conditions including acne, pimples, eczema, psoriasis and more.

Using the information provided in this book, carefully choose the essential oils that meet your needs and preferences. Always keep safety precautions in mind. Learn more about your preferred essential oils and experiment with your own blends.

Introduction – Essential Oils

Commonly called essences, essential oils are natural oils extracted from plants. Their liquid form is usually distilled using water or steam from plant elements such as the bark, roots, leaves, stems, and flowers. While most of them have a clear color, there are some like lemongrass, orange, and patchouli that are yellow or amber in color. Since they are highly concentrated, a little amount can go a long way. People can benefit from essential oils through inhalation or direct application to the skin or hair.

Unlike actual oils, essential oils don't contain fatty acids. Instead, they are highly concentrated plant elements possessing potent qualities for medicinal and cosmetic purposes. Essential oils are the soul, or life force, of a plant. Their high contents of anti-viral, anti-fungal, and anti-bacterial properties make them effective for cleaning the home and treating cuts or wounds. Since they are small in molecular size, the hair and skin absorb them well, which makes them a perfect addition to hair and skin care items designed to nourish, soften, and heal. Several scientific studies show that some essential oils like rosemary help relax the brain, which allows it to function in top condition.

What Makes Essential Oils Different from Fragrance Oils?

Essential oils are entirely different from fragrance oils. Even if the fragrance oils are tagged as natural fragrances, they are still made from synthetic ingredients that are unnatural. On the other hand, essential oils are completely natural. Because of this reason, they cannot be patented. In turn, it limits the scientific study of these oils tremendously. Nevertheless, many things that we need to know about these oils have been passed from generation to generation through thousands of decades of personal experimentation and use.

How to Store Essential Oils and Safety Tips

Essential oils do not become stale. However, a number of them oxidize in time and lose their therapeutic properties. Some can lose their aroma and therapeutic benefits as quickly as six months. On the other hand, certain essential oils mature with age.

In general, all types of essential oils benefit from proper storage. This avoids deterioration and protects their aroma and therapeutic properties. To keep them away from sunlight, it's best to store them in cobalt blue or other dark glass containers. Avoid placing them in plastic containers because essential oils will react with plastic and ruin their therapeutic properties. Make sure they are kept in cool places away from the sunlight.

There are a variety of essential oils and each have their own benefits. People who like using them as an alternative to prescribed medications should take extra precautions when using them. If you are pregnant or nursing, avoid some essential oils, such as sage, rosemary, nutmeg, lemon, jasmine, ginger, clove, clary sage, cinnamon, chamomile and cedar wood. Since they are highly concentrated and potent, they should be diluted properly to enjoy their maximum benefits. Avoid eye contact with the oils. Perform a skin test before using the essential oils to avoid irritation. Avoid taking them internally, especially eucalyptus and wintergreen oils. Most importantly, keep these oils away from the reach of children.

Benefits of Essential Oils

Skin Benefits

- *Certain essential oils relieve dry and irritated skin, which makes them suitable for those suffering from eczema and psoriasis.*

- *Some have deodorizing properties to keep skin smelling clean and fresh.*

- *Others have anti-oxidant properties for tightening and rejuvenating aging skin.*

- *Some essential oils are best suited for treating dry skin.*

- *Certain essential oils are used as an astringent for oily skin.*

- *Some essential oils used for toning the skin are also used for treating acne, wounds, burns and insect bites.*

Hair Benefits

- *Certain essential oils help stimulate the scalp to reduce oiliness, minimize dandruff and stimulate hair growth.*

- *Other oils add shine to dull hair.*

- *Some essential oils strengthen and moisturize hair.*

Nails

- *Some essential oils are potent enough to kill fungi that cause infections of the fingernails and toenails.*

- *Other oils strengthen brittle nails.*

- *Some oils promote nail growth.*

Eyes

- *Some essential oils have an anti-inflammatory effect that can address dark circles when applied slightly below the eyes.*

- *Others can reduce puffiness and swelling under the eyes.*

- *Some can be used as a moisturizer for smoothing under-eye skin.*

Additional Benefits

- *Some essential oils are used in massages to promote complete relaxation, relieve headaches, sore muscles and menstrual cramps.*

- *Others use fragrant essential oils in a diffuser as a natural air purifier.*

- *Inhalation of some essential oils stimulates deep sleep. They also relieve colds and sore throats.*

Helpful Tips for Using Essential Oils

1. Dilute essential oils before applying them to the skin.

2. If it is your first time using an essential oil, do a skin patch first.

3. When skin becomes irritated, you should cease using the essential oil.

4. Be careful not to get any essential oil into the eyes or mucus membranes.

5. *Always wash your hands after coming in contact with pure essential oils.*

Most Effective and Commonly Used Essential Oils

Basil

In the past, basil essential oil was used for digestion, addressing respiratory problems, treating fevers and healing snake bites. Today, it is more popularly known for its anti-inflammatory and anti-spasmodic properties. It is a rich source of vitamins A and K, calcium, potassium and other minerals. Its leaves also contain anti-microbial and anti-oxidant properties, which make it a perfect solution for treating skin infections.

Additionally, Basil is also used as anti-bacterial,

anti-viral, antiseptic, decongestant and stimulant. Though the basil essential oil has many benefits, it is most beneficial to the cardiovascular, skeletal and muscular body systems. It can be inhaled directly or diffused into the air. It can be applied straight to the skin or used with coconut oil, which is ideal for sensitive and young skin.

Chamomile

Chamomile oil has a sedative effect that induces sleep. It is often served with lemon or honey to enhance its effect. Chamomile has been found to have an anxiolytic or anti-anxiety component that lessens stress, insomnia and anxiety. It also contains Alpha- bisabolol, which is used as an antiseptic, and it has anti-inflammatory characteristics. Chamomile has been used topically for inflammations caused by hemorrhoids. The chemical components of chamomile extract have an anti-hyperglycemic agent, anti-inflammatory, anti-genotoxic and anti-cancer properties. Chamomile oil cannot be used by women who are pregnant or delivering because it can promote uterine contraction. Chamomile oil also causes a drug to drug interaction when used with other medications.

Eucalyptus Oil

This essential oil is made from eucalyptus leaves with numerous benefits as a medication or treatment. Its primary active component is cineol or eucalyptol, which provides a camphoraceous aroma. It also has expectorant and antiseptic properties. It has been used as a pharmaceutical remedy, antiseptic solution for wounds, repellent, flavoring and fragrance. It can treat the symptoms of influenza, fever, burns, ringworms, bronchitis, cough and colds. The medication comes in inhalants, vapor rubs, ointments and lozenges. It also stimulates the immune system response in the body. Eucalyptus has also been used as flavoring for baked goods, meat products and sugar confectioners. It's also used in soaps, lotions, detergent and perfumes to add fragrance.

Evening Primrose Oil

The primary element in evening primrose oil is gamma-linolenic acid or GLA. This essential fatty acid is required by the body for healthy growth and development. It has a wide range of both therapeutic and preventive qualities; herbalists recommend it for preventing diseases and maintaining youth. It's used to treat skin disorders like acne, eczema and psoriasis. It also treats rheumatoid arthritis, osteoporosis, multiple sclerosis, heart disease, high cholesterol, Alzheimer's disease, alcoholism and schizophrenia.

It relieves asthma, nerve damage associated with diabetes, weight loss, whooping cough and gastrointestinal disorders such as irritable bowel syndrome, peptic ulcer disease and ulcerative colitis. It's suitable for treating diseases with women's health. It prevents high blood pressure during pregnancy, late deliveries and shortens labor. Women experiencing PMS can use this oil. It helps prevent breast pain and reduces the unfavorable symptoms brought on by menopause.

Hemp Seed Oil

Hemp seed oil is a good source of both LNA or Omega 3 and LA or Omega 6 in a balanced proportion. This oil has been used to treat conditions involving deficiencies in LA and LNA. LNA helps keep the skin smooth, speed the body's healing process and increase the body's stamina. It helps to increase vitality, reduce inflammation, reduce water retention, minimize platelet stickiness and reduce blood pressure. The oil enhances immune functions, reduces pain and swelling of arthritis, reverses pre-menstrual syndrome, and treats bacterial infections.

Jasmine

Jasmine flowers contain high amounts of etheric oil. The flower contains benzilic acetate, benzilic alcohol, linalcohol, jasmine and indole. All of these substances contribute to the aphrodisiac property of jasmine oil. Aside from its aphrodisiac property, jasmine also aids in the improvement of digestion, weight loss and toxin elimination. It helps boosts metabolism and improve blood circulation.

Jasmine oil is a commonly used oil in aromatherapy. It's recommended for physical pain. Moreover, it has a powerful antiseptic, tonic and sedative effect, which helps treat breathing difficulties, nervous debility and coughing.

Jojoba Oil

Jojoba oil is extracted from the seeds of simmondsia chinensis plants. Unrefined oil from jojoba plants is a clear golden substance with a nutty smell. Though it has a similar appearance with to other vegetable oils, its chemical composition resembles outlawed sperm whale oil. It is composed of 40-42 carbon chain length esters composed of fatty alcohols and monounsaturated fatty acids. This pure material is made of all-wax esters and less than 1 percent triglyceride content. It also contains Vitamin E and phospholipids, which are beneficial to the skin and hair.

It has been used as an additive to beauty products such as lotions, moisturizers, shampoos and conditioners. Thanks to a component in the oil, it gives skin and hair deep moisturizing treatments. It has also been used as an antifungal medication for mildew fungi. It can also be used to replace whale oil. Other uses of jojoba essential oil are a foot and hand softener, after shaving cream, cuticle oil, massage and bath oil and eye and face makeup remover.

Lavender

Due to its versatility, lavender is a popular essential oil. Among its most influential chemical compounds are lavandulyl acetate, geraniol and linalool. These natural chemical compounds provide it with a light, fresh aroma. When inhaled, it allows you to relax, unwind and alleviate stress. It also has antiseptic properties for treating colds and the flu. It is best used for those who are suffering from migraines and asthma. It's highly recommended for its skin benefits, treating skin problems like acne, wounds, insect bites, burns, psoriasis and stings. When used for massages, it helps relieve pain caused by rheumatism, arthritis and sore muscles. Since it is an adaptogen, lavender can help the body adapt to imbalances. Moreover, it boosts stamina.

Myrrh

Myrrh essential oil contains formic acid, acetic acid, heerabolene, m-cresol, eugenol, cuminaldehyde, limonene, cadinene, a-pinene and other sesquiterpenes that are responsible for its medicinal properties. It has been used in almost all of the potions in Ayurveda medicine. It is known for several health benefits. When used in vaporizers, myrrh can treat coughs, colds and bronchitis. When used as a mouthwash, it helps to prevent dental infections. If used as a massage oil or added to bath water, it enhances the skin's condition and treats infections in women. Using a cold compress, it treats sores and wounds. Myrrh essential oil treats skin ulcers when mixed with lotions. Its fragrance refreshes and rejuvenates the senses.

Olive Oil

Olive oil extracts are obtained from grinding whole olives. It contains saturated fats and is commonly used for cooking, pharmaceutical ingredients and making soaps. It contains 14 mg, or 93 percent, Vitamin E, which helps in skin care. In ancient Egypt, olive oil was used as a home remedy for skin care. It's mixed with beeswax and used as a cleanser, moisturizing cream and anti-fungal cream agent. In Greece, it is used as a topical muscle relaxant for sports injuries.

Studies have little evidence of olive oil curing acne pimples, but a promising result from studies shows olive fruit contains squalene. Squalene has been used as an antioxidant and moisturizer. Another study also reported evidence that olive oil mixed with beeswax and honey can relieve skin from rashes, dermatitis, eczema and other skin diseases infected by staphylococcus aureus and candida albicans. Olive oil is also used to help reduce levels of blood cholesterol and obesity. Studies show a regular intake of olive oil decreases blood pressure. It is also used in patients with diabetes to help maintain blood sugar levels and insulin sensitivity.

Peppermint

Peppermint essential oil has high contents of menthol. It also contains methyl esters, menthone and other compounds like pinene, caryophyllene, eucalyptol, pulegone and limonene. These constituents activate the receptors in the mucosal tissues and skin.

Its strong, mental smell makes peppermint an essential oil popularly used in aromatherapy.

Since it is cool and refreshing, this essential oil is best for stimulating the mind and improving concentration. It helps relieve headaches, migraines, anxiety, stress, asthma, dry cough, bronchitis, cholera, pneumonia and tuberculosis. It relieves pain caused by aching feet, aching muscles, toothache, rheumatism and painful menstrual periods. It benefits the skin by relieving irritation, itchiness, redness, sunburn and skin. It can treat acne, scabies, dermatitis and ringworm. Peppermint oil stimulates bile secretion and the gall bladder. For this reason, it is effective in treating ailments such as colic, dyspepsia, nausea, flatulence and spastic colon.

Rose

This valuable essential oil requires numerous pounds of petals to produce just one ounce of oil. It has several properties that contribute to its health benefits. Its major components include Phenyl Graniol, Pheneylmenthyl Acetate, Phenyl Acetaldehyde, Nonanal, Nonanol, nerol, Methyl Eugenol, Stearpoten, Farnesol, Ethanol, Eugenol, Citronellyl Acetate, Carvone, Citral and Citronellol.

It functions as an anti-depressant fighting depression and relieving anxiety. As an antiseptic, it treats wounds and prevents infection. Since it relieves spasms, it's an antispasmodic. Moreover, it has anti-viral properties that shield the body from viral infections. Rose essential oil has anti-bacterial properties that treat bacteria-causing diseases like typhoid, cholera and diarrhea. It works as an astringent to strengthen gums and hair, tone and lift skin and address other signs of aging.

Rosemary

Rosemary oil has numerous natural properties, which help with skin and hair care. It works great for aromatherapy. Its chemical components include beta-caryophyllene, limonene, camphene, thujone, camphor, bornyl acetate, terpinen-4-ol, alpha-terpineol, linalol, borneol, pinene and cineole.

With its refreshing and powerful herbal smell, rosemary is one of the essential oils widely used in aromatherapy. It has numerous therapeutic properties. As an analgesic, it's effective in relieving headaches and muscle and joint pain. It helps lower blood cholesterol levels in those who are hypertensive. With its strong diuretic properties, it allows uric acid and other wastes to be eliminated through urine. It has anti-bacterial and astringent properties, which make it effective in treating dental conditions leading to healthy teeth and gums. It strengthens hair and promotes growth. It's great for skin care, reducing acne, wrinkles and sun spots. It provides relief from colds and allergies. Furthermore, it boosts concentration, enhances memory and reduces anxiety.

Sandalwood

It is an essential oil extracted from steam distillation of chopped heartwood in a sandalwood tree. Its main chemical components include santalene, santyl acetate and santalol. Also, it has high content of sesquiterpenes, a chemical element stimulating the brain's pineal gland. This helps increase melatonin production, which promotes sleep and boosts the immune system.

The oil of this plant has been used in perfumes, sacred unguents and additives for cosmetics. It has a sweet, woody, warm scent. It is also used as an antiseptic for wounds and internal medications. Its antimicrobial compound is suitable for clearing the skin of black heads, spots and acne. The oil must be diluted first before applying to the skin due to its strong components. The plant has properties used as antidepressants, antiviral, immune system stimulant, bronchial dilator, anti-tumoral, tonic and a sedative. It's also good for aromatherapy, which is good for relaxing the mind and body.

Tea Tree Oil

Tea tree oil has been used as a traditional medicine. Often used as an inhalant, its chemical constituents include a-terpineol, terpinen-4-ol, linalool, terpinolene, p-cymene, y-terpinene, 8-cineole, limonene, a-terpinene, a-phellandrene, myrcene, sabinene, b-pinene and a-pinene.

It's pale yellow or pale gold color has a camphor scent. Suggestions indicate that tea tree oil has a lot of medical properties as a topical remedy. It can be used as an anti-fungal, antibacterial, antiviral and antiseptic for wounds. It can also treat acne, congested noses, destroy head lice, body odor, dandruff, sinusitis and sunburn. Moreover, tea tree oil is also used as a cleaning agent for dish-washing liquids, laundry soaps and bathroom cleaners. It can also be used as an insect repellent for hiking and camping.

Thyme

Over the centuries, thyme has been used for numerous purposes. In fact, it was used in ancient Rome to treat melancholy. It was also added to alcoholic beverages and cheese. Ancient Greeks used thyme as incense. Thyme also has some culinary uses. Thyme essential oil is added to dishes like stews, soups and casseroles. Also, it is used for medicinal purposes in antiseptic ointments. Thyme was also added to toothpastes and soaps to improve teeth, gum and skin health.

Its main active element is thymol, which is an antiseptic that is effective against fungi and other infections. It also contains essential compounds such as linalool, borneol, myrcene and p- Cymene.

Witch Hazel

Witch hazel is also known as spotted alder or winter bloom. This flowering shrub is commonly found in North America. Its essential oil has been used as a medical astringent for quite some time. Witch hazel provides numerous benefits. Its main constituents include phenolics, particularly tannins, which are used to help aid in healing skin problems.

It can be used for treating acne. This also helps reduce eye puffiness from lack of sleep or crying. The leaves and twigs of witch hazel can be soaked in hot water and made into a tea to cure sore throat. Other benefits of witch hazel include a reduction in varicose veins, healing of a bruise, cleansing a wound, relieving itch, refreshing the skin, refining the pores and sealing in moisture in the skin.

Few Oils Not Good for the Skin

Many people, particularly those who are conscious of the way they look, apply numerous ingredients to their skin every day. Of these ingredients, several are known carcinogens and toxins, which are generally absorbed by the skin and into the body where they are stored and cause adverse effects to the body. Some of these ingredients are oils.

Mineral Oil

Mineral oil is a common ingredient in numerous personal care products from foundation to moisturizers, hair products and lip balm. Mineral oil acts as a moisturizer to the extent that it keeps portions of the skin moist. Although most moisturizers are composed of essential nutrients that care for the aging and fragile facial skin, mineral oil has no nutrients.

Mineral oil seals off the skin, averting it from breathing. It attracts the required moisture in the cells, which are deep inside the skin. This can cause collagen break down, slow cell renewal and damage of the connective tissue.

Petroleum Oil

One of the most damaging ingredients normally found in skin care products is petroleum oil. This kind of oil was revealed to block the ability of the skin to moisturize itself, resulting in chapped and dry skin. Petroleum oils are identified to block skin pores, which can aggravate skin conditions such as acne and dermatitis and stop the skin from excreting toxins through its pores.

Hydrogenated Oil

Hydrogenated oils are usually healthy in their natural state, but are immediately turned into toxins because of the processing they go through. When hydrogenated oils reach the skin cells without sufficient essential fatty acids, the cells are forced to use the destructive hydrogenated oil. The existence of hydrogenated oils in the skin cell walls averts nutrients from entering into the skin cells. At the same time, it is letting in microbes, viruses and pathogens into the skin. Hydrogenated oil prevents waste matter from exiting the skin cells. With the waste material trapped inside the skin cells and the nutrients placed out of the skin cells, the cells usually mutate or die. This can lead to tumors, cancer or other serious medical issues.

Emu Oil

Emu oil, which can be found in numerous skin topical treatments and lotions, can result in skin irritation when applied to the skin. Most emu oil products are composed of multiple ingredients and chemicals, which further enhances the growing danger of an allergic reaction.

Moreover, emu oil shouldn't be used for treating open wounds because it contains elements with acidic qualities.

What is Carrier Oil?

Carrier oils are a type of vegetable oil often used as a base for diluting essential oils before applying to the skin. Essential oils are too concentrated to be applied to the skin. This type of oil is named a carrier oils because it carries the scent of the essential oil to the skin where it is absorbed.

Basically, carrier oils are vegetable oils derived from fatty parts of the plant. The usual parts used are kernels, seeds and nuts.

Why Carrier Oils Are Considered Important?

Some people wonder why there is a need to combine essential oils with carrier oils when they are both oils. Essential oils are typically undiluted and highly concentrated. When the oils are applied to the skin, it can cause severe irritation and result in an allergic reaction on sensitive skin. Carrier oils are important because they are used to dilute essential oils before application. Carrier oils carry the essential oils to the skin.

The Aroma of the Carrier Oils

Carrier oils have a different aroma, but some are odorless. Most carrier oils have a faint, sweet, nutty aroma. There are times when the aroma of carrier oils becomes strong and bitter, which is because the oil is rancid.

Different Types of Carrier Oils

There are different kinds of carrier oils. Each type of carrier oil offers different effects when it comes to therapeutic characteristics and properties. When choosing carrier oils, one must consider the therapeutic benefit being sought.

Below are some of the best carrier oils commonly used today:

Sweet Almond Oil

This carrier oil is affordable and all-purpose carrier oil today with a light, sweet, nutty aroma. The body absorbs the oil in a semi-quick manner.

Aside from being used on the skin, this oil can also work wonders for your hair. It nourishes the hair, making it stronger, longer and thicker, adding shine to it and controls hair fall. Almond oil is also used in massage therapy or aromatherapy.

Grapeseed Oil

This carrier oil is an all-purpose oil that can be used in a wide array of applications like skin care and massage. It has a relatively short shelf life compared to other types of carrier oils. When applied to the skin, it leaves a glossy film on the skin's surface.

Macadamia Oil

This carrier oil is sought for its natural anti-inflammatory properties. It's considered a good option for massage applications. When applied, it leaves an oily film on the skin.

Apricot Kernel Oil

This carrier oil has a semi-oily texture. Its characteristics make it a good choice for massage applications.

Avocado Oil

This carrier oil is best used for nourishing hair and skin. It is rich in essential trace minerals and Vitamin A. Due to its aroma and thick consistency, this carrier oil is used in low ratio blends and formulas.

Sunflower Oil

Sunflower oil is an all-purpose carrier oil with a faint, sweet aroma. It is a good choice for massage applications since it doesn't leave an oily residue and is easily absorbed by the skin.

Olive Oil

This carrier oil has an oily texture, heavy viscosity and strong aroma. When it comes to skin care and aroma therapy, this oil is not as widely used.

Pomegranate Oil

This carrier oil is an effective emollient. Moreover, it's also rich in anti-oxidants due to its polyphenol content. It is best used for dry, aging and irritated skin. It provides protection from free radicals and helps destroy the cells that cause cancer.

Hazelnut Oil

This carrier oil penetrates well into the skin and is a good choice for those who have oily skin. It's also used in aroma therapy applications, ranging from skin care to massage.

Cranberry Seed Oil

This carrier oil offers a balanced mixture of omega 3, 6 and 9 fatty acids. It is also rich in Vitamin E and A. It helps nourish the skin and reduce the signs and symptoms of aging. This oil helps treat scarring, eczema and psoriasis.

Fractionated Coconut Oil

Coconut oil is commonly used for hair and skin. Coconut oil is considered one of the best oils for hair. It can help hair grow healthy by reducing protein loss and adding shine. It also helps keep the hair free from dandruff and lice. Moreover, coconut oil has been used for massage therapy and is best used for dry skin.

These benefits are attributed to the presence of caprylic acid, capric acid and lauric acid in the coconut oil. It also contains soothing, anti-bacterial, anti-fungal, anti-oxidant, and anti-microbial properties.

Natural Ingredients for Body Care

Skin benefits from natural ingredients like essential oils extracted from plants. They contain nutrients that deliver proper skin health and balance. Even though they are potent enough on their own, blending them with other essential oils provides a synergistic effect unless done incorrectly.

Avocado

Avocado contains Vitamins A, B (B1 & B2), C, D and E. It's also rich in fatty acids, pantothenic acid and proteins. This makes the oils suitable for people with dry, sensitive skin and those with eczema and psoriasis. If this ingredient is mixed incorrectly with other oils, it may cause more harm than good to the skin.

Carrot Seed

One of the most overlooked essential oils, carrot seed adds suppleness to the skin, rejuvenating and stimulating it. At the same time, it addresses skin problems like eczema and psoriasis. It also fights age spots and wrinkles.

Clary Sage

It has astringent, anti-bacterial, anti-inflammatory and antiseptic properties that make this essential oil ideal for oily and acne-prone skin. It helps treat eczema, psoriasis and boils. It also has the ability to reduce wrinkles because it promotes regeneration of skin cells.

Geranium

Geranium is helpful in skin care due to its ability to treat acne, burns, dermatitis, eczema, lice and wounds. It's best for oily and mature skin. It firms loose skin and prevents varicose veins.

Lemongrass

Lemongrass, which has a refreshing aroma, is used to cleanse skin and moisturize due to its mild astringent properties. It helps skin eliminate waste and toxins. It also has the ability to rejuvenate tired, sagging skin. It works best when used alone.

Ylang-Ylang

This essential oil is known for balancing the skin. Ylang-Ylang essential oil has the ability to control sebum secretion. It soothes and balances extra dry or extra oily skin.

Blending Essential Oils

When blending essential oils, it is important to consider their appropriate volumes. Exceeding the required maximum amount can cause adverse skin reactions. Storage is another important consideration. When not stored properly, essential oils can easily oxidize and blend with other ingredients.

Skin and Hair Types

Since essential oils are not the same and have different chemical components, they may have different effects when used by different individuals. What is good for one person may not be appropriate for another. It's best to know the type of skin and hair you have before using essential oils. Below are simple ways to determine the type of skin and hair a person has:

Determine your Skin Type

As the largest organ in the human body, this soft covering serves as a barrier from diseases, prevents extreme water loss, regulates temperature, produces vitamin D and is responsible for sensation. Having beautiful skin depends on a person`s diet and skin care regime.

Normal / Combination Skin

70 percent of the total population across the world have normal or combination skin. This type of skin is the least problematic and easy to maintain.

Characteristics

- No traces of oil
- Vibrant, supple and elastic
- Clean, smooth and good blood circulation
- Healthy and glowing complexion

How to determine

- Slightly oily in the T-zone area of the face, while cheek areas are dry.
- Dry patchy spots found anywhere on the body.
- Pores in the forehead and cheeks may be larger than other parts of the face.

Oily Skin

This is the most problematic type of skin. Excessive oil on the skin may be caused by various changes, which may include hormonal changes, weather and temperature changes and genetics.

Characteristics
- larger pores and break outs due to excessive oil in the face
- looks greasy, thick and shiny
- prone to aging and wrinkle formation
- prone to blackheads, pimple, acne and other skin blemishes

How to determine
- The T-zone (from forehead, nose and chin) is shiny and greasy.
- It leaves oil marks or spots on dermal paper.

- Excessive oil in the face, regardless of whether the weather or temperature is fair.

Dry Skin

This type of skin requires special care. Most women experience dry skin when they reach 35 years of age. When exposed to drying factors, the skin cracks, peels and becomes irritated and itchy. Dry skin may be caused by genetic factors, weather, aging, heat, medications and application of skin care products.

Characteristics

- tight, dry and scaly
- less elastic
- visible lines and pores
- red patches
- flaking

How to determine

- Dermal paper appears clean with a few oil spots.

- Upon washing the face, skin feels tight, dry and has a pale tone.

Sensitive Skin

This skin type is very fragile and requires specialized skin care. Certain cosmetic products irritate the skin easily.

Characteristics

- thin and delicate
- fine pores

How to determine

- If a cosmetic product is not suitable for the skin, it results in itching, dryness, redness and burning of the skin.

Determine your Hair Type

The hair is considered a person's crowning glory. Since it can either make or break a person's physical appearance, the hair is one of the most delicate parts of the body. Every person has his or her own type of hair, which can be easy or difficult to manage.

Fine Hair

This hair is naturally shiny and is damaged. It needs proper care.

Normal Hair

This hair is not thick or thin. Also referred to as the medium hair type, it falls between fine hair and coarse hair and is easy to style.

Coarse Hair

This hair usually feels rough, strong, dry, wiry and wild. It requires deep conditioning to keep it shiny and easy to handle.

Ways to determine the type of hair

a) Wash air dry hair. Observe the time it takes for your hair to dry. If it takes ½ hour to dry, the hair might be fine and thin. If it takes more than an hour, the hair is probably thick. Upon drying, if the hair is smooth and naturally silky, the hair is a fine type. If the hair is dry, wiry, damaged and wild, the hair could be a coarse type.

b) Pull a strand of hair and place it on a piece of paper to observe. If the hair cannot be easily seen or felt by the finger on top of the paper, the hair type is fine. If the hair is easily visible on the paper and is not wiry to the touch, the hair type is normal or medium. If the hair is easily seen on the paper and feels wiry, the hair type is coarse.

Essential Oils for Skin Care

Anti-Aging Recipes

Different types of skin can benefit from the natural essential oils. Using them regularly and properly will not only allow you to manage skin problems, but also help enhance your skin tone and elasticity. It will result in a more youthful appearance.

Jojoba Oil Anti-Aging Serum for Dry Skin

This anti-aging serum helps reduce the appearance of wrinkles and fine lines. Its main ingredient is jojoba oil, which moisturizes the skin and provides lasting hydration without clogging the skin's pores. This essential oil is comparable to natural skin oils in humans. For this reason, it easily penetrates the skin. When combined with other essential oils and compounds, it nourishes, moisturizes and softens dry, mature skin. Jojoba essential oil helps control acne and sebum production in the scalp. It's great for skin care because of its soothing and balancing properties. It helps fade dark spots and even skin tone.

Ingredients:

½ tsp. Vitamin E

1 oz. pomegranate seed oil

2 oz. rosehip seed oil

10-20 drops jojoba oil

Procedure:

· In a clean bottle, mix all ingredients. Gently shake the bottle until all ingredients are blended well. Seal the bottle and store in a cool, dark place. Do not refrigerate the serum.

· After cleansing the face, apply a pea size

amount of the serum to the affected area. Massage until it is completely absorbed.

· Use twice daily. During daytime, use a sun block.

Evening Primrose Anti-Aging Facial Cream for Oily Skin

This anti-aging facial cream reduces the signs of aging, increases elastin levels, promotes production of collagen and assists cell regeneration. Its main ingredient, evening primrose oil, contains high amounts of essential fatty acids, which promotes healthy skin. This results in a youthful, firmer and smoother skin tone with enhanced elasticity. It helps treat oily skin.

Ingredients:

3 tsp. evening primrose oil

1.5 tsp. beeswax pastilles

3 tsp. apricot kernel oil

1 tsp. coconut oil

2 tsp. jojoba oil

8-10 tsp. rose-water

Procedure:

· Mix all ingredients, except rose water, in a boiler or stainless pan. On low heat, allow wax to melt for five to eight minutes. Stir the ingredients well.

· Remove pan from heat and stir in rose water slowly.

· Place mixture in a 2.5 oz. jar and refrigerate until set.

· Apply twice daily, morning and evening, under eyes and other affected areas.

Almond Oil Anti-Aging Facial Mask for Normal Skin

This anti-aging facial mask helps reduce the appearance and development of wrinkles. It's more effective when combined with daily facials. Its main ingredient, almond oil, is rich in Vitamin E and moisturizing properties. Also, it works great for all skin types. With the mixture of other essential oils and compounds, this anti-aging mask helps improve the skin's complexion and retain its glow.

Ingredients:

1 tsp. Almond oil

1 tbsp. extra virgin Olive oil

2 tbsp. Oatmeal

1/2 cup Buttermilk

Procedure:

- In a boiler, mix oatmeal and buttermilk.
- Once the oatmeal is soft, add olive oil and almond oil to the mixture.
- Remove from heat and set aside. Allow mixture to cool for 5-10 minutes.
- Apply mask to a clean face and neck using your fingertips. Avoid getting the mixture into your eyes and lips.
- Leave the mask on your face for 25 to 30 minutes and relax.
- Rinse with cool water. Avoid using soap.
- Pat skin dry with a clean towel and apply an anti-aging toner and moisturizer.

Lavender Rose Anti-Aging Face Cleanser for Sensitive Skin

This face cleanser is a great addition to your facial regimen. Not only will it thoroughly cleanse the skin, but it also maintains the skins glow and health. Its main ingredients are rose and lavender essential oils, which are effective in treating mature skin. Combined with other necessary elements, the oils help reduce the appearance of fine lines and wrinkles. Moreover, the oils are safe for sensitive skin.

Ingredients:

5 drops rose essential oil

5 drops geranium essential oil

10 drops lavender essential oil

6 tbsp. grapeseed oil

1 tbsp. brown sugar (optional)

Procedure:

· Pour all oils into a clean, dark glass container or bottle.

· Gently shake the bottle to allow the oils to blend well.

· Store the bottle in a cool place, but avoid putting it in the refrigerator.

· Before each use, shake the bottle and apply to the face using a circular massage.

· Rinse with warm water. Pat skin dry with a clean cloth.

· If you want to use the cleanser as a facial scrub, simply add brown sugar before applying it to the skin.

Essential Oils for Facial and Body Scrub

Essential oils are now used as a facial and body scrub giving the skin vitality and cleansing. The essential oils are made from natural ingredients with a minimal to no undesirable effects to sensitive skin.

Eucalyptus Sugar Scrub for Oily skin

This scrub works great for oily skin. It helps remove dead skin cells, leaving the skin fresh and glowing. Its main ingredient is eucalyptus oil, which provides a refreshing feeling.

Ingredients:

Half cup white refined sugar

¼ cup coconut oil

2-3 ml eucalyptus

Procedure:

· Mix coconut oil and sugar in a boiler. Heat until it reaches a thick consistency.

· Remove from heat and add eucalyptus oil to the mixture.

· Apply mixture to the body using a gentle circular massage for five minutes.

· Rinse properly and pat skin dry.

Chamomile Lavender Sugar Scrub for Combination skin

With its sedative and relaxing properties, this scrub relaxes skin from daily stress, exfoliates dead skin and induces a good night sleep. Its main ingredients are lavender and chamomile, which promote glowing and healthy skin.

Ingredients:

2 cups salt

1 cup sea salt

½ cup baking soda

4 ml. lavender oil

2 ml. chamomile oil

30 ml. almond oil

Procedure:

· Mix ingredients in a boiler on low heat.

· After five minutes, add essential oils and stir

until the mixture is thick.

- Remove from heat and allow mixture to cool.
- Apply scrub to your body.
- Rinse thoroughly.

Tea Tree Scrub for Normal skin

Tea Tree scrub contains tea tree essential oils, which exfoliate and moisturize the skin. It deeply cleanses the pores, leaving a healthy, glowing and younger looking skin.

Ingredients:

1/3 cup white sugar

1 tbsp. sea mineral salt

1 tbsp. baking soda

15 drops tea tree oil

Olive oil extracts

Procedure:

· In a pot, warm all ingredients on low heat.

· Stir until mixture thickens.

· Remove from heat and allow mixture to cool.

- Apply in a circular motion.
- Rinse with warm water and pat skin dry.

Essential Oils for Facial Care

If you're searching for a pure and all-natural material to restore young and radiant skin tones, essential oils might be the solution you seek. Essential oils are frequently used to treat certain skin conditions, as well as to maintain healthy skin.

Jasmine Facial Wash for Dry Skin

This facial wash cleanses skin impurities and tones irritated, dry and sensitive skin. It contains jasmine oil, which helps increase the skin's elasticity. It is often used to treat stretch marks and minimize scarring.

Ingredients:

¼ cup milk

¼ cup cream

2 tbsp. jasmine essential oil

Procedure:

· Heat ¼ cup milk, ¼ cup cream, and two tablespoons jasmine oil in a saucepan.

· Let sit for two hours.

· Pour into a sterilized jar and keep in the refrigerator.

· Apply to face in circular movements.

· Rinse thoroughly.

Witch hazel facial toner tightens the skin and draws out oil and other impurities that clog pores. It contains witch hazel essential oil, which has anti-inflammatory properties that aid in preventing skin inflammation from acne. When combined with other essential ingredients, the toner provides a revitalizing effect on skin and promotes a balance of moisture.

Ingredients:

2 cups distilled water

3 tsp. dried leaves of bee balm

2 tbsp. witch hazel essential oil

1 tbsp. lime juice

1 tbsp. lemon juice

Procedure:

· Boil two cups water and place three teaspoons dried leaves of bee balm into water.

· Let sit until the leaves are golden brown.

· Remove dried bee balm leaves and place tea into a jar and let cool.

· Afterwards, add two tablespoons witch hazel, one tablespoon lime juice and one tablespoon lemon juice.

· Shake jar gently until ingredients are blended well.

· Use as a facial toner twice daily for best results.

Coconut Facial Nourishing Treatment for Combination Skin

This facial nourishing treatment contains high moisture retaining properties, which provide a soothing and softening effect on skin. It helps protect skin from dryness and itchiness, while keeping it soft and smooth.

Ingredients:

1 drop Ylang-Ylang essential oil

5 drops orange oil

6 drops rose oil

1 oz. pure coconut essential oil

Procedure:

· Blend one drop Ylang- Ylang oil, five drops orange oil and six drops rose oil into one ounce pure coconut oil in an amber or dark colored bottle.

· Apply mixture to face using gentle massage.

· Perfect for applying after sun exposure and as a daily skin nourishing treat.

Rose Lavender Toner for Normal Skin

Rose lavender toner contains essential fatty acids, Vitamin A and Vitamin C. It's ideal for protecting your skin and increasing cell turnover. It also contains relaxing properties, which calm and refreshen the skin.

Ingredients:

8 oz. distilled water

2 drops lavender essential oil

1 drop palmarosa oil

1 drop rose essential oil

Procedure:

· Pour eight ounces distilled water into a clean container.

· Add two drops lavender oil, one drop palmarosa oil and one drop rose oil.

· Mix thoroughly.

· Apply toner to skin after cleansing.

· Shake well before use.

Essential Oils for Face Mask

Skin experiences a lot of stress from weather conditions and physical activities. Since the face is the most exposed part of the body, it receives a lot of chemical ingredients in make-up and beauty products that may contain harsh chemicals. Using essential oils, homemade facial mask recipes can be used to give the face a spa worthy relaxation and rejuvenation for a glowing and youthful skin appearance. It's best to know what skin type is suitable with what essential oil to ensure effectiveness of the recipe.

Hemp Seed Facial Mask for Dry skin

Moisturize and maintain the elasticity of your skin with a hemp seed facial mask. It deeply nourishes the skin and helps remove wrinkles and fine lines caused by dry skin.

Ingredients:

¼ cup hemp seed oil

½ avocado

Procedure:

· Peel the avocado and place half of it in the blender.

· If desired, add fragrance oil and blend thoroughly.

· Scoop blended mixture into bowl. Add hemp seed oil and stir thoroughly.

· Place hemp seed and avocado mixture in microwave and heat for 20 seconds.

· Stir mixture and set aside to cool.

· Wash face and pat dry. Apply facial mask and leave on for 30 minutes.

· Remove mask and rinse face thoroughly with warm water.

Tea Tree – Aloe Vera Gel Facial Mask for Oily Skin

Pamper your skin with tea tree and aloe vera gel facial mask. It contains anti-bacterial properties, which help in treating acne, pimples and blemishes caused by excessive oil in the face. It's best used for facial cleansing due to its deep cleaning and ability to close pores.

Ingredients:

1 teaspoon tea tree oil

1 ounce aloe vera gel

3 teaspoons water

Procedure:

· Heat ingredients in a pan.

· Stir until consistency thickens.

· Remove from heat and allow to cool.

· Wash face and apply mixture to the face.

· Leave on for 30 minutes and rinse thoroughly.

Rosemary Mud Facial Mask for Combination skin

Not only will the mask help remove deep dirt trapped inside the pores, but it also helps regenerate skin. It contains essential compounds, which help moisturize and nourish the skin.

Ingredients:

1 teaspoon pure moor mud

1 teaspoon rosemary oil

2 teaspoons thistle oil

½ cup water

Procedure:

· Boil moor mud in a hot pan until it reaches a paste consistency.

· Mix all remaining ingredients until dissolved evenly.

· Remove hot pan from fire and set aside to

cool.

· Wash face with water and pat dry.

· Apply mud evenly to face and leave for 20 minutes.

· Rinse thoroughly and pat dry.

Lavender Facial Mask for Normal skin

This facial mask helps you achieve smooth skin. It contains anti-bacterial properties, which prevent skin infections and irritations. It also helps the skin fight against free-radicals and aging.

Ingredients:

2 tablespoons pure honey

3 drops lavender oil

1 teaspoon hot water

Procedure:

· Heat all ingredients in a small saucepan until the consistency is thick.

· Remove from heat and allow the mixture to cool.

· Wash face with warm water and pat dry.

· Apply mask evenly to the face.

· Leave on for 30 minutes.

· Rinse thoroughly and pat dry.

Essential Oils for Hair Care

Like the skin, hair experiences stressors every day. It's one of the main parts of the body frequently damaged from excessive heat from the sun and chemical agents. Countless hair treatments and products produced on the market promise to bring life back to hair. Essential oils are highly recommended for all hair types. You can do these hair treatments at home. It's always best to know the type of essential oil that will work best for your type of hair.

Sandalwood Conditioning for Dry Hair
Sandalwood conditioner moisturizes and nourishes the roots of the hair. It deep conditions hair from the roots to the tips.

Ingredients:

5 tsp. castor oil

5 tsp. jojoba oil

20 drops sandalwood essential oil

1 egg yolk

Procedure:

· Combine 5 tsp. castor oil, 5 tsp. jojoba oil, 20 drops sandalwood oil and one egg yolk in a pan on low heat.

· Stir the mixture to a thick consistency.

· Remove from heat and allow the mixture to cool.

· Apply to the hair as a conditioner and leave it for about 20 minutes.

· Rinse hair thoroughly and air dry.

Basil shampoo for Oily Hair

Basil shampoo works great for oily hair. It contains essential elements, which slow down the oil production of the sebaceous gland.

Ingredients:

120 ml liquid castile soap

½ teaspoon vegetable glycerin

¼ teaspoon vitamin E

30 ml aloe vera

5 drops basil oil

Procedure:

· Mix 120 ml liquid castile soap, ½ teaspoon vegetable glycerin, ¼ teaspoon vitamin E, 30 ml aloe vera and 5 drops basil oil.

· Pour mixture into a tinted glass bottle and cover tightly.

· Label properly and store.

· Use as a hair shampoo.

Thyme Conditioning for Oily Hair

Thyme contains a conditioning agent that keeps hair healthy and soft.

Ingredients:

5 ml. vegetable oil

1 tbsp. emulsifying wax

1 tsp. grape seed oil

1 capsule Vitamin E

½ cup distilled water

Procedure:

· Mix 5 ml. vegetable oil, 1 tbsp. emulsifying wax and 1 tsp. grape seed oil into a boiler.

· Slowly melt the wax on low heat.

· Remove the boiler from the stove and add 1 Vitamin E capsule.

· In a separate pot, heat ½ cup distilled water.

· After heating the water, remove the pot from the fire and slowly pour water into the oil mixture. Stir the mixture well until the consistency is smooth.

- Set it aside and let it cool.
- Pour into an airtight container.
- Label properly and store.
- Use as a hair conditioning treatment.

Rosemary Anti-Dandruff Shampoo

Rosemary anti-dandruff shampoo cleans the pores of the scalp. It contains ingredients that keep the hair hydrated and dandruff free.

Ingredients:

¼ cup distilled water

1 cup rosemary oil extract

15 drops camphor oil

Procedure:

· Boil ¼ cup distilled water and 1 cup rosemary oil extract in a pot.

· Fully boil the mixture and set it aside for 6 hours.

· After 6 hours, add 15 drops camphor oil and stir.

· Apply the shampoo to the hair and massage your head for five minutes.

· Wash hair thoroughly and towel dry.

Tea Tree Oil Scalp Treatment for Oily Hair

Tea tree oil scalp treatment gives you a minty fresh feeling and reduces the activity of the sebaceous gland producing excessive oil.

Ingredients:

1 cup olive oil

15 drops tea tree essential oil

Procedure:

· Warm 1 cup olive oil into a double boiler for 5 minutes. Do not boil the oil.

· Remove the olive oil from heat and add 15 drops tea tree oil extract.

· Mix the oils evenly and allow the mixture to cool.

· Apply treatment to the hair and scalp.

· Wrap the head for 15 minutes.

· Rinse hair thoroughly and dry.

Chamomile Shampoo for Normal Hair

Chamomile shampoo relaxes the head and promotes proper blood circulation that keeps the hair healthy.

Ingredients:

1 ¼ cup hot water

¼ cup chamomile essential oil

1 ¼ cup chopped soap

1 tbsp. glycerin

Procedure:

· Place 1 ¼ cup hot water in a bowl and add ¼ cup chamomile oil extract.

· Set the mixture aside for 15 minutes.

· Combine 1 ¼ cup chopped soap into the chamomile mixture.

· Let the mixture stand for 5 minutes.

- Add 1 tbsp. glycerin and stir until properly blended.
- Pour mixture into tinted glass bottle.
- Close and label properly.
- Use to shampoo the hair.

Rose Conditioning Treatment for Normal Hair

Rose conditioning treatment contains nutrients that help maintain and promote healthy hair.

Ingredients:

1 egg yolk

3 tbsp. eucalyptus oil

1 squeezed lemon

5 drops cedar wood oil

3 drops rose oil

Procedure:

· Mix one egg yolk, 3 tbsp. eucalyptus oil, 1 squeezed lemon, 5 drops cedar wood oil and 3 drops of rose oil in a bowl.

· Apply mixture to the hair and leave it for 5 minutes.

· Rinse hair thoroughly and dry.

Eucalyptus Anti-Dandruff Shampoo for Normal Hair

Eucalyptus anti-dandruff shampoo relaxes the head and nourishes hair strands and the scalp to make it healthy.

Ingredients:

1 tablespoon apple cider vinegar

15 drops eucalyptus oil

10 drops grape seed oil

2 ounces mild natural shampoo

2 ounces water

Procedure:

· Heat 1 tablespoon apple cider vinegar, 15 drops eucalyptus oil, 10 drops grape seed oil, 2 ounces mild natural shampoo and 2 ounces water.

· Stir until mixture is thick and even.

- Remove from heat and set aside to cool.
- Use as an antidandruff shampoo.

Lavender Scalp Treatment for Normal Hair

Lavender scalp treatment promotes a relaxing and fresh feeling to the scalp. It reduces the activity of the sebaceous gland responsible for producing excessive oil.

Ingredients:

1 cup olive oil

15 drops lavender essential oil

1 egg yolk

Procedure:

· Warm 1 cup olive oil in a double boiler for five minutes. Do not boil the oil.

· Remove olive oil from heat and add 15 drops lavender oil extract.

· Mix the oils evenly.

· Add one egg yolk and stir thoroughly. Set

aside to cool.

- Apply treatment to the hair and scalp.
- Wrap the head for 15 minutes.
- Rinse hair thoroughly and dry.

Essential Oils for a Relaxing Massage

Massage therapy using essential oils boosts overall wellness. It provides relief for pain in the muscles, joints and other systems. It balances the body, mind and spirit. Some essential oils are best used during summer and winter due to their cooling and warming properties, respectively.

Head Massage

A head massage is an effective remedy for anxiety, depression, insomnia and stress. Aside from providing relaxation, it helps improve concentration.

Lavender and Chamomile Summer Massage Recipe

A lavender and chamomile massage recipe provides cooling and soothing effects to the body, which makes it great to use during summer months. It contains essential properties, which help to relax and cool stressed and tired muscles.

Ingredients:

12 drops lavender

12 drops chamomile essential oil

¼ teaspoon Vitamin E

4 ounces infusion oil (½ part chamomile flowers, ½ part lavender buds and 2 parts oil)

Procedure:

· Mix all ingredients in a clean, amber bottle.

· Use it for a summer massage.

Rose Winter Massage Recipe

Rose winter massage oil recipe is a great stress reliever. It contains properties that promote warmth and relaxation to the body, which makes it perfect for winter massage therapies.

Ingredients:

5 drops rose essential oil

½ cup extra virgin coconut oil

Procedure:

· Mix all ingredients in a jar and keep in a cool temperature.

· Use to massage the head and scalp.

Head Massage Technique

The best way to massage the head is with the balls of the fingertips. Using circular motions and moderate pressure, the massage starts from the sides and works up toward the top of the head.

Neck Massage

Neck pain can interfere with daily activities. It can be relieved by massaging with essential oils.

Peppermint Summer Massage Recipe

Peppermint massage oil contains menthol, which cools and relieves neck pain. Its cooling properties make it great for summer massages.

Ingredients:

2 drops peppermint
almond oil

Procedure:

· Combine 2 drops of peppermint with a little almond oil.
· Rub into the neck to relieve tension.

Rosemary Winter Massage Recipe

Rosemary massage oil has the ability to warm muscles in the neck and improve blood flow. The warming effect makes it great for winter massage therapies.

Ingredients:

5 drops rosemary oil

jojoba or almond oil

Procedure:

· In your palms, mix 5 drops of rosemary oil with a little jojoba or almond oil.

· Apply this mixture to your neck, and then, gently massage it.

· Wrap a thin scarf around your neck to prolong the effect.

Neck Massage Technique

This can be done in a sitting or standing position. Apply massage oil, and then, slide the fingers along the line between the shoulder and the base of the head. Bend your neck towards the other shoulder and repeat. Do this on the opposite shoulder. Grab the base of the neck with your fingers and pull up. Do it again along the length of the neck.

Shoulder Massage

Eucalyptus Summer Massage Recipe

This summer massage recipe relaxes tight and stressed muscles. Its eucalyptus ingredient provides cooling and soothing effects to the affected area. These effects make this recipe a perfect ointment for summer massages.

Ingredients:

60 drops eucalyptus essential oil

8 ounces grape seed oil

4 ounces organic walnut oil

2 sprigs dried rosemary

Procedure:

- Blend all ingredients in a blender.
- Pour the mixture in a pump bottle.
- Use this to massage tired shoulders.

Jasmine-Ginger Winter Massage Recipe

This winter massage recipe helps reduce inflammation and improve blood circulation. It increases the body's temperature, which makes it the perfect ointment for winter massage treatments.

Ingredients:

10 teaspoons ginger (carrier oil)

6 drops ginger essential oil

4 drops jasmine essential oil

Procedure:

· Combine all ingredients in a bottle.

· Use for winter massages.

Shoulder Massage Technique

Place the essential oil in the palm of the hands. Rub hands together. Place hands onto the shoulders and carefully rub the skin. Let it be for 40 minutes before wiping it away.

Back Massage

Lemon-Lavender Summer Massage Recipe

Lavender relieves stress and promotes sleep. With its fresh fragrance, lemon can uplift the spirit. It also contains refreshing properties, which are good for summer massage therapy.

Ingredients:

2 drops lavender

2 drops eucalyptus

1 drop lemon

20 ml. carrier oil

Procedure:

- Combine all ingredients in a bottle.
- Use to massage the back.

Sandalwood Winter Massage Recipe

Sandalwood provides relaxation in all applications. When mixed with almond oil, sandalwood warms up the body temperature making it suitable for winter massages.

Ingredients:

8 teaspoons almond oil

6 drops sandalwood essential oil

Procedure:

· Mix all ingredients in a bottle.

· Use formula for a winter massage.

Back Massage Technique

Give a slow stroke along the length of the back. Let the hands walk up the spine, applying pressure for a few moments in every location.

With the thumb moving in a circular motion, apply medium pressure on the area above the hips to both sides of the spine. Knead the shoulder and neck areas and gently pinch them.

Leg Massage

A leg massage relaxes the legs, relieves pain and prevents cellulite formation.

Lavender-Almond Summer Massage Recipe

Lavender has calming properties to help legs relax. It lowers the body temperature, which makes it great for use in summer.

Ingredients:

5-10 drops lavender oil

2 tbsp. almond oil

Procedure:

- Mix all ingredients in a bottle.
- Store in a cool place and use to massage legs.

Rosemary-Peppermint Winter Massage Recipe

Combining rosemary and peppermint helps to soothe muscle aches. It also contains properties, which regulate blood circulation and make the body feel warm. This makes it ideal for winter massages.

Ingredients:

10 tsp. grape seed oil (carrier oil)

2 drops peppermint

3 drops eucalyptus

4 drops rosemary

Procedure:

· Mix all ingredients in a bowl.

· Use for leg massage.

Massage technique

Following the shape of the legs, apply pressure beginning with the foot all the way to the thigh. Firmly stroke the thighs. Use knuckles to massage the upper thigh. Massage the knees in a circular motion with your fingertips. Tighten grip on calf muscles, and then, pull away from the leg bone.

Toes Massage

Toes are part of the foot. When massaged, they provide relief to the entire body.

Chamomile-Lavender Summer Massage Recipe

Lavender has both antibacterial and calming properties, while chamomile has antibacterial and antiallergenic properties that are beneficial for toe health. Both oils have soothing properties, which cool down the body. This is perfect for summer massage therapy.

Ingredients:

3 drops lavender

1 drop chamomile essential oil

2 teaspoons olive oil

Procedure:

· Mix all ingredients in a bottle.

· Store in a cool temperature and use for a toe massage.

Olive-Peppermint Winter Massage Recipe

Peppermint is strong and minty, which refreshes and relieves achy toes. Olive stimulates circulation, which increases the body temperature. They work great for winter massages.

Ingredients:

Olive oil (carrier oil)

5 drops peppermint

6 drops eucalyptus essential oils

Procedure:

· Pour olive oil (carrier oil) into a bowl.

· Add 5 drops peppermint and 6 drops eucalyptus essential oils.

· Mix thoroughly to use as massage oil.

Massage Technique

Pour massage oil into your hands. Rub them together. Massage toes by gliding the thumb between each tendon. From the base of the toe, firmly squeeze through each tip.

Essential Oils for Lip

Unlike other parts of the body, the lips don't have sebaceous glands to keep them moisturized. For this reason, they easily become chapped and dry. Thanks to essential oils, your lips stay protected and moisturized.

Lip Balm

The skin on lips is thinner than the rest of the face. It easily peels when dry. During colder months, it gets worse. To keep them well-hydrated, it is best to use a lip balm. By using a lip balm, your lips are moisturized and look plump. A lip balm made with essential oils is more beneficial because it is all-natural and doesn't contain harsh ingredients that can cause harm. It has a unique flavor and scent. It also contains the same benefits provided by the essential oils it is made with.

Coconut Oil Lip Balm

Ingredients:

1 tablespoon coconut oil

1 tablespoon olive oil

1 tablespoon beeswax

Procedure:

· Blend coconut oil, olive oil and beeswax.
· Heat the mixture in a double broiler.
· Allow the essential oils and wax to melt together.
· Mix well. Pour into a container. Let cool before use.

Coconut Oil Benefits

Coconut oil is not only beneficial to health but also to beauty. It helps moisturize, nourish and cool the skin. It has a sweet scent and a long shelf life. These qualities make it ideal for use as an ingredient in lip balms.

Mint Flavored Tea Tree Lip Balm

Ingredients:

2 tablespoons jojoba oil

3 drops peppermint essential oil

2 drops tea tree essential oil

2 teaspoons beeswax

Procedure:

· Mix jojoba and beeswax in a metal container.
· Heat until wax is completely melted and fully integrated with the jojoba.
· Remove from heat. Add peppermint and tea tree essential oils.

Peppermint Benefits

Peppermint is known for its fresh menthol smell and scent, which gives a minty flavor to lip balms. It helps to smooth and soften dry, cracked lips. It also cools sunburned lips.

Tea Tree Benefits

Tea tree is effective in treating dry, chapped lips with its healing properties.

Essential Oils for Dark Circles under the Eyes
The skin surrounding the eyes is the thinnest skin layer in the face. It's prone to puffing from allergies, crying, colds and infection. These conditions cause an accumulation of water around the eye bags leaving it loose and dark when it subsides. Due to modern studies, essential oils are now recommended to fix flaws under the eyes. They are safe, effective and budget-friendly remedies. They are suitable for all types of weather and can be applied at home.

Eye Miracle Cream Recipe
Ingredients:
2-3 drops almond oil
Facial cream (preferred)

Procedure:

· Mix the almond oil into the facial cream. Almond oil can also be used alone.

· Gently pat the mixture onto the skin under the eyes.

· It is best applied before bedtime to allow the almond oil time to absorb into the skin overnight.

Benefits of Almond Oil

It contains a moisturizing agent that helps in rejuvenate the skin under the eyes. It also contains vitamin A and palmitic acid, or a fatty acid, which nourishes the skin. Almond oil hydrates the skin, making it look younger and fresh. It relaxes the muscles and promotes circulation around the eyes.

Witch Hazel Soothing Eye Gel Recipe

Ingredients:

1 tsp. cucumber juice

1 tbsp. Aloe Vera gel

1 tbsp. witch hazel essential oil

¼ tsp. corn starch

Procedure:

· Mix cucumber juice, aloe vera gel and corn starch in a sauce span.

· Heat ingredients for one minute. Do not boil the ingredients.

· Remove pan from heat after one minute.

· Add witch hazel essential oil and stir the mixture thoroughly.

· Set the mixture aside to cool down. Consistency must be a jelly or gel like.

· Scoop the mixture out of the pan and into an

airtight jar.

· Dab fingers into the gel and apply a small amount under the eyes.

· Leave it on for 15 minutes to promote blood circulation. Leaving it for more than 30 minutes may cause rebound effects.

· Rinse the eye gently and pat dry.

Benefits of Witch Hazel Oil

Studies show that witch hazel oil has the ability to contract and shrink blood vessels, which causes dark circles under the eyes. It contains an anti-inflammatory agent, Chyrish, which promotes proper blood circulation under the eyes. It may work well if incorporated with other essential oils such as eucalyptus oil, which gives a minty feeling.

Essential Oils for Nail Care

A person's overall health is often reflected on his or her nails. Nail growth can differ from one person to another. Healthy nails grow faster. They are smoother and rarely show any flaws. Essential oils provide proper nail care for those with nail imperfections.

Nourishing Nails Recipe

Ingredients:

20 drops lavender

10 drops lemon

1 tablespoon almond

1 tablespoon jojoba

Procedure:

· Drop essential oils little by little into a dark colored glass bottle with a dropper top.

· Then, include the base oils. Close the bottle with its dropper top.

· Shake forcefully for two minutes. This allows all the ingredients to

   blend and warm to your body temperature.

· Leave the bottle in a dark area, 60-80° F, for 24 hours to allow the essential oils to work synergistically with one another.

· Place a drop on each nail and massage with a soft cloth.

· Do this every night. Dispose of the solution after six months.

Lavender

Lavender is not only soothing, but it can also stop the growth of common types of fungi that cause infections to the skin and nails. When a fungus infection of a nail is left untreated, it can spread to other nails. Using this on a regular basis will not only treat nail fungus, but it will also prevent infections in the future.

Lemon

Nails benefit from lemon. It whitens the nails and stimulates healthy nail growth.

Almond

Almond, which is a natural emollient, can restore moisture to your nails. When massaged into the nails, it makes them look shinier.

Jojoba

Jojoba essential oil can repair both nails and hands. It provides enough moisture for nails to grow stronger. When used regularly, nails will absorb Vitamin E. This helps enhance nail quality.

Castor Oil Soak

Ingredients:

3 to 4 tablespoons castor oil

10 drops myrrh oil

Procedure:

· Place ingredients in a small glass bowl. Mix thoroughly using a spoon.

· Cover the bowl. For every treatment, use 1 tablespoon of the mixture. Place bowl in hot water until the warmth is bearable.

· Allow clean fingers to soak in the solution for 5 to 10 minutes. This will soften the nails and cuticles.

· Let your fingers dry. Gently push cuticles with a small piece of cloth. Use this for buffing nails as well.

· Use a moisturizer to further soften your hands.

· You can do this three times per week.

· Keep the remaining solution in the refrigerator and dispose of it when it is a month old.

Myrrh

This essential oil is a very potent antioxidant. By adding about 3 drops of Myrrh to the base of the nail, it can strengthen brittle nails and promote healthy nail growth.

Essential Oil Kits for Keeps

People who are new to essential oils can get started by trying them in smaller glass bottles, which are available in kits for office, travel and everyday use. You can try different kinds of essential oils without spending a lot on a couple of the bigger bottles. These kits come in handy whenever and wherever the user needs the essential oils.

At Home

Just like a first aid kit, a basic kit should contain at least three small containers of essential oils for basic needs.

Lavender

Lavender is a multi-functional oil, which can be handy at home. It serves as an antibiotic, antiseptic, antidepressant, detoxifier and sedative. Since it can promote healing and prevent scarring, it's best applied when you get burns. It also stimulates sleep.

Tea tree

Tea tree is potent enough to treat acne, athlete's foot, toothaches, infections and sunburn.

Peppermint

Peppermint has special antiseptic and anti-inflammatory properties that treat conditions ranging from indigestion to migraines and rheumatism.

At Office

This kit should contain essential oils for addressing some of the ailments that are common in workplaces.

Eucalyptus

Eucalyptus relieves symptoms of colds and flu. It also helps to alleviate headaches. Eucalyptus oil functions as a natural sanitizer by adding a few drops to water.

Peppermint

Stomach disorders can happen to anyone, but this can be addressed with peppermint as it has anti-inflammatory properties to effectively relieve heartburn and stomach ulcers. Moreover, peppermint essential oil can treat allergies by reducing body inflammation.

Chamomile

Chamomile essential oil can allow a person to relax and stay focused at work.

For Travelling

A travel kit should have the essential oils that you may need during a trip. They normally include oils for travel sickness, jet lag, insect bites and sunburn. These essential oils will allow you to sleep well, feel comfortable and enjoy the trip.

For Insect Bites: lavender, tea tree and aloe vera

Lavender is a natural insect repellent, but it is also useful for healing insect bites. It provides quick relief for itching.

Tea tree helps reduce itching and the sting caused by insect bites.

Peppermint oil keeps mosquitoes away. In case you get bit, this can help stop the swelling and allow it to disappear immediately.

For Jet-lag: eucalyptus, chamomile and peppermint

Eucalyptus awakens the senses with its sweet and fruity aroma. You can apply it topically or use it aromatically.

Chamomile tea has chamomilla to soothe frayed nerves and emotional stress caused by jet lag.

Peppermint Oil – When inhaled, the aroma of peppermint oil can alleviate jet lag. This essential oil is a natural stimulant for relieving mental fatigue and stress.

For Sanitizing: thyme, rosemary and eucalyptus

Thyme essential oil has several active principles for promoting health and preventing diseases. When added to a vaporizer, it will disinfect the air. To fight against food-borne salmonella, a few drops can be added to water used to clean washing boards and kitchen boards.

Rosemary oil can be mixed with a few drops of vegetable oil to clean small wounds. It disinfects water by adding a few drops to it. It also disinfects surfaces when used as a household cleaner.

Eucalyptus has natural disinfectant properties that make it a suitable replacement for harsh chemical cleansers.

For Moisturizing: coconut, almond and jojoba

Coconut is popularly known for its skin softening and moisturizing properties. Its effectiveness in treating dry, scaly skin is comparable to mineral oil. However, unlike mineral oil, coconut oil does not clog pores.

Almond oil is very light, yet it is filled with important fatty acids and moisturizing properties.

Jojoba oil has the ability to reduce wrinkles and stretch marks as it deeply moisturizes the skin.

Final Words

I hope you must have not only enjoyed this book but also tried few recipes for your skin and hair type. If you want to let others know about your experience, please post your valuable and constructive reviews. Your feedback matters and it really does make a difference.

I would greatly appreciate your comment because your review is going to help me improve and update my work. If you found any error or anything you suggest to change or add in this, do let me know at satenyada@gmail.com and I promise a quick personal response.

Your review is going to make a true experience for other readers and help them make their buying decision easier. If you'd like to leave a review then all you need to do is go to review section of book and click on "Write a customer review".